Come Smile With Me

From the heart of a polio survivor

'Life is a bowl of cherries, not
all of them are ripe,
and some are rotten'

By

Peter Thwaites

ISBN: 1-4140-2481-9 (e-book)
ISBN: 1-4140-2480-0 (Paperback)
ISBN: 1-4140-2479-7 (Dust Jacket)

This book is printed on acid free paper.

1stBooks - rev. 11/25/03

Preface

I am a survivor of the Polio epidemic in the UK during the early 1950's and over the past five years have been experiencing the demoralising affects of Post Polio Syndrome (PPS)

I have written this short autobiography as a means to easing my way out of a period of particular tiredness and anxiety, and was suggested by my Psychologist. I hope that it makes you smile and maybe cry, although this is definitely not my foremost intention.

Many of the episodes are drawn directly from memory at the moment of writing and so, over the passage of time, occasionally; events may be betrayed slightly differently than they should. I have, however, endeavoured to be frankly honest in my depiction of the last fifty years of my life and must stress at this point that I regret nothing. I have, for the most part thoroughly enjoyed my life and truthfully hope that there are many years and experiences still to be encountered.

Dedicated to my mum and dad, without whom I would never have survived, thanks.

Episode 1

1949, the war has been over now for almost four years. Although the rationing of some basic items has still to be discarded, much of the population of the United Kingdom are beginning to rebuild their lives amidst the death, destruction and confusion that still remains, if not in fact, in memories, thoughts, and nightmares.

Worthing, a thriving seaside resort with pier, promenade and miles of golden sand is situated on the South Coast of Britain betwixt Brighton and Littlehampton and is one of the UK's major attractions during the summer months. Even during the winter season, the pier is an ideal place for the catching of the occasional flounder, bass, and if you are really unlucky an eel or two.

Young families can often be seen standing on the pier's timber decking, crabbing, with small metal containers filled to the brim with struggling crabs of all sizes, (not all complete with the requisite number of legs) trying to make a quick escape back to the ocean. Not to worry though, for at the end of the day, all and sundry are tipped unceremoniously into the sea, before the weary children head towards the nearest fish and chip shop arguing about who had caught the largest crab.

Much of the older section of Worthing, especially close to the town centre itself, contains many fine Victorian and Edwardian detached houses. With the ending of the war, finances are poor and instead of these refined properties falling into disrepair many discerning owners have converted them into small bedsits. Many of these are not self contained with the occupiers sharing facilities with other residents.

It is almost spring, the 9th March, and in one of these small but comfortable bedsits, I am born, kicking and screaming, to fantastic parents brought together by the fortunes of the war some two years earlier. The owner of the bedsits, an eccentric and affectionate elderly lady, of much wisdom and experience, appears over the top of my new cot, cigarette ash dropping on to the soft pristine covers like gently falling snow, and wisps of white and blue smoke floating serenely across the room. My mother and father show concern and I am quickly moved out of harms way by the local midwife who has attended the home birth, so common these days.

I weigh in at a very reasonable 8lb and have all of the necessary equipment for a young lad, so life is good. My hair is a bit thin on top, a precursor for later life, and judging by the various noises that I can produce nothing wrong in the voice department.

Mum and dad are deliciously proud, and at every opportunity I am displayed to my cooing relatives.

In a very short space of time I am able to create a whole range of directions that must be acted upon, such as I need a drink, a meal would be good, how about a bit of burping, oh, and by the way, this nappy is decidedly wet.

Growing up is an exciting business and I enjoy every moment, the walks in the park, the pram rides, bird song, the wind, rain, sleep, meal times, being washed, and that wonderful hazy smell of talcum powder. Oh what a time I can have with that—it is amazing how far such a small amount can travel. I am an expert at being sick, as well, I can target the point of contact precisely, and as for timing, well!.

1951 should be another fine year, but disaster; suddenly I have a competitor, a brother. Obviously I am in charge as the biggest and eldest, but he seems to be a bit slow on the uptake, and it takes a long time before he accepts this inevitable fact. However we get there in the end, and after all, he is quite nice, really.

I am a lot more independent now, and my brother, who seems awfully slow, is still crawling about on all fours like a cat. I am certain that I never had to do that. Still, he is an ideal collaborator for the occasional prank on mum and dad, although even if it isn't always my fault I am continually getting the blame.

Worthing, like many larger towns throughout the UK is attracting many new residents year by year and with the majority of these as young families, the local authority is steadily increasing it's housing stock. One such development is in Durrington, which lies to the North West of Worthing, and here hundreds of new houses are being built to house the increasing population.

My family is gradually growing and as it is getting a bit cramped where we are, mum and dad apply to the local authority for a council house, and after a short wait we are all off to live in a marvellous two-storey house in Durrington.

Moving day is a nightmare for my brother and I, as we can't find our toys anywhere, but as we have our very own bedroom, things are certainly looking up.

What a wonderful new home this is, everybody is very happy, we even have our own toilet, outside in the yard, and when I sit on the seat, I can see under the door right down to the end of our garden. Mind you, in the winter, the wind seems to find its way everywhere. The floor gets a bit wet when it rains too, but it is ours, and we don't have to share it with anyone. I am making lots of new friends and all in all, life is grand.

We have our own fireplace with a real fire, and each Christmas my brother and I hang up our stockings. Father Christmas has never ever forgotten us, and there are always loads of exciting parcels to unwrap. This year we have an enormous Christmas tree—fantastic! It is taller than my brother, or I, and is covered with beautiful sparkling and twinkling coloured balls. I can see myself if I look at one of the balls and I am always smiling. There are also strings of silver and gold that seem to wind their way up the tree, and at the very top, there is a pretty fairy holding a tiny wand. I know that she is wishing us all a very happy Christmas.

I can hear people singing carols, and smell delicious aromas of chocolate, wood smoke, cigars, pine needles, and turkey. I wish this could last forever.

Christmas passes and over the next couple of years, I get all of the usual childhood illnesses, measles, chicken pox, etc., "better to get them all now—whilst you're young"—I'm reminded, whilst buried under my bedclothes feeling ill and totally depressed. I don't want to be young if it means being ill all of the time.

There are a lot of young families living near us, and one of my mates lives next right door. He is not really a friend because he is a bit rough and always in trouble, but occasionally we have some fun together. Today, however he has a really bad cold, and something wrong with his foot so we don't do much, except build a small camp at the bottom of my garden. We have both got toy guns and play cowboys and Indians. I'm always the cowboy because I have the best gun. We are completely lost in our own world of baddies, goodies, camps, friendly fights and lots of mud and dirt. Suddenly A—Tishhhhhhhhhhhhhh—ooo and I'm drenched. I don't like this part of the game. I'm going back indoors in the dry. This is not fun anymore and I am not going to play with him again until his cold goes away.

Throughout life it is strange how you take things for granted—but I had always thought that once you mastered the technique, ascending and descending stairs is a real cinch. Until today, that is. For some reason, after successfully mastering the top two treads on the way down to breakfast for 'tapping egg' and marmite soldiers, the remainder becomes a blur and the next thing I remember I am laying flat out on the hallway floor. Not a pretty sight, and very sore. Pride is a very tender thing, but even more so is your backside, and it would appear that I have landed on it.

Out comes the usual axiom "If you don't take more care, and end up breaking your leg, don't come running to me". Do parents actually listen to what they are saying—they must think we are all too young to understand.

Anyway, back to my soreness and to add insult to injury I have now to contend with my younger brother's not so witty comments. Still the marmite soldiers are good, and I have soon forgotten about the incident completely. I am a bit wary on the stairs today and hang on to the handrail going up and down. Occasionally I feel a bit wobbly in the garden, but come on; I'm only four.

About a couple of weeks later it happens again. This time I am fortunately half way up, or down (I can't remember which), but whatever, my bum makes contact with every step on the way down, until the inevitable happens and I make contact with the floor—OUCH. This time it is not funny, and I forget my age, and burst into tears. Look, I am four years old, man of the house, (after my dad, of course), and falling down stairs does absolutely nothing for my 'street cred'. If my friends ever get to hear of this.

On this occasion, I am also feeling a bit unwell, hot, and sweaty, and there is a strange and worrying sensation in my left leg. A bit like 'pins and needles'. It is a good thing that I am not a bit older, or I might begin to panic, but I will leave this up to my mum, she is really good at it.

Like all great adventures they come and they go, and if I forget all the times lately that I have fallen over, or inexplicably dropped something, I am getting on well, until today.

Early morning, the sun is beginning to rise and there are noises out in the street. People are beginning to start their day and all is well with the world.

I can hear dad downstairs making the morning tea. Everyday he would get up at about 6.30, make us all a cup of tea and bring it up stairs to our beds with a slice of bread and margarine. We couldn't afford biscuits, although mum did manage to get a bag of broken biscuits from 'Isteds', a general provisions store in the town centre. Dad worked for them for a while.

Getting up in the morning was never my strong point, and the tea and bread made it a lot more tolerable. This morning, however, I have a bit of a problem. I can't move. Not just my arms or legs, but nothing, absolutely nothing. Everything has gone numb—I can't even wriggle my toes—this is not funny, extremely frightening and I am now beginning to the panic. Nobody is going to believe me. I feel really ill. I have a hot, sweaty feeling that appears to move around my body. My head feels as though it is about to explode, and I can actually hear my own pulse.

I have told dad, and he looks a bit shocked, now it's mum's turn. I gather that dad has gone to fetch the Doctor, and all I can do now is wait, literally! The room is beginning to spin round and I feel that I am floating just off the top of my bed. I feel that I am about to be violently sick and I'm right. Mum is rushing around with towels and flannels, although it is becoming increasingly difficult to make out anyone in the room. I just know that it is my mum. My brother is fast asleep.

This is desperate—I can't move a thing, and it is no good prodding me about, I can't feel it either. I don't feel anything. For goodness sake, Doctor, what is wrong? It is exactly like being in a dream, more likely a nightmare, when you want to move, but you can't. I am not able to control any part of me, even talking is becoming difficult—come on you lot—sort it out. Surely dad knows what to do?

This ambulance is fast, and I can make out the bell—I wish I wasn't so scared—I might be able to enjoy this. I wonder where I am going. I can make out mum sitting on the bed opposite mine, but I don't know where dad is, or my brother. I feel really sleepy but the bells keep waking me up. We seem to be going miles and miles...

I have never felt so dreadful. My head still hurts and my throat is swollen and sore. I can see that I am in a strange bed, in a sort of goldfish bowl, with tubes coming out of me from everywhere. I can see mum through the glass standing in a very pretty area filled with flowers of every type and colour. I wonder why she is not in here with me; I could really do with a cuddle right now. There is someone coming inside the 'bowl', they are dressed in some sort of white gown and wearing a mask—they look very strange, and somewhat concerned. Maybe I am a bit of a problem to them—I don't mean to be. I still can't move anything—I am very scared, "please help me". Even I can't hear that, so there is no chance of anyone else hearing me—what can I do?—Very sleepy..................

Mum and dad are in here with me, they've got the same clothes on as the other person, and they are wearing masks, but I can hear them and recognise them so I must be getting better. I feel a bit better, more relaxed. My head doesn't ache quite so much, but I can still hear my pulse.

There's another man standing close to dad. He is quite small with grey hair and looks very old, and appears to be wearing a white collar, and carrying a book. None of them look very happy to see me—I wish I could touch mum—but I can't move. Dad looks really sad. "Come on Dad, I'll be back home soon"—I wish I didn't feel so slee....................

Strange. It is beautiful. I am standing on the shore of a gently flowing river, which in front of me is a magnificent shade of blue with gentle white waves lapping against my feet. All around me are trees and flowers of every imaginable colour swaying quietly in the warm summer sun. I can see the sunlight reflecting like shafts of diamonds on the top of the water. I feel truly happy, content and peaceful. The light blue sky has several miniature fluffy clouds that are being blown around by the warm summer's breeze. I am at ease. Through the summer haze I can see a small wooden rowing boat coming towards me from the opposite bank. There doesn't appear to be any movement but it is definitely getting closer, and standing in the centre of the boat is the most beautiful man I have ever seen. His face is full of gentleness and caring, with his arms held outstretched towards me. He is tenderly dressed in a combination of light brown and a white flowing robe with a half raised hood of similar material, and almost appears to be floating.

I find myself walking slowly towards him, and as I get closer, with a voice like that of angels, he is telling me that I am far too early to take the boat with him and that I must return home. I have many friends waiting and praying for me. His tone was soft and yet commanding, full of compassion and love.

Mum is back and she seems to be very happy, I can't see dad or my brother. I am in a strange kind of metal tube, lying on my back, with a mirror just above my face. This is really odd. I still can't move anything on my own, but I can feel my chest going up and down, and there is this sort of steam sound. Maybe I am in a steam engine, but why?

Hey, everything is upside down, how on earth am I going to drink anything? I get it; I drink using a long bendy straw, wow that tastes good. It seems like ages since I had a drink.

Well I am certainly getting around—I am back in the goldfish bowl and there seems to be a group of Doctors with my mum and dad. None of them are wearing those dreadful masks anymore. Maybe I am going home soon. I think I am sitting up, but I am not sure how I got like this, mind you it is a lot better than lying on my back.

I don't remember much about the last few months, except that I was allowed to go home and had to wear callipers. I learnt to walk all over again and managed to begin using my arms and hands. I could even go to the toilet on my own. It feels like ages ago that I was doing that. My home is a wonderful place, I love my mum and dad, and even my little brother. I don't want to leave them all behind ever again. It made me very sad.

When I was a lot older I was told that I had caught Infantile Paralysis or Polio as it is more commonly known. I had also actually *died* for a couple of minutes. The Doctors had told mum and dad that if I survive the night, it was very unlikely that I would ever sit up again, and to walk again was out of the question. No wonder they looked unhappy. What traumas we have to bear as parents! Mum and dad had been surrounded by loving friends and relations, and on the night that I almost crossed the river, had spent the entire night praying for my recovery in a small chapel nearby. The many prayers had been answered.

The vision and sensations experienced that night are as vivid today, as they were at the time. I have no doubt that what I experienced, for me, was real and I have never had any reason to doubt this. I don't know what it means; I am not sure what I believe. I can only let you, the reader, come to your own conclusions.

It is likely that I contracted polio the day my mate from next door was playing in our camp. He had been banned from going out of doors that day. He had a very mild form of polio that affected his right foot. The virus was transferred to me through the simplest of things. The sneeze from his cold.

Episode 2

I am a big six now and progressing very
well, considering the doctors' prognosis. I
am still having physiotherapy, mainly on my
legs that don't want to work too well. I
wear a sort of brace during the day, but
mum can take it off when I am in bed, so
that's good. My friends don't seem to
notice that I am wearing anything
different, which really helps me get
through the days, and at night I feel
normal. I have noticed that one of my legs
is thinner than the other, but this will
get better I am sure. Mum and dad don't
talk about it much. I don't want to be
special, just normal. Perhaps I am normal
already?

Today is not going to be a nice day as I am
going to see my physiotherapist at the town
clinic. Mum takes me on the back of her
bike and it is quite a way so she is
exhausted when we arrive. I have to sit in

a miserable sort of waiting area packed with other people with all sorts of illnesses and problems. One of the many doors leading off this area goes to the school dentist. I dread going through that door, it makes my skin crawl and I will do anything to avoid it. The dentist seems reasonably human, but his nurse—I think she hates kids, and especially me. She reminds me of the wicked stepmother in Sleeping Beauty. She scares me with her look and makes me feel very frightened.

Oh, it's my turn to see the physio now, so I go into a funny smelling room. There is a long bench against a wall, an old swivel chair, a long desk like table covered with piles of paper, and loads of files. I like my physio. I have been seeing her for a long time now, and we have got to know each other. She is very kind and gentle and seems to listen to what I am saying. I know that most doctors don't. She tells me to take off my socks and shoes, which I do, and place my feet in a bowl of water. There is a sort of transformer box on the table and some wires that she attaches to one of my legs. Wow... That stings—I get a sort of electric shock in my foot, which makes my whole foot twitch. I am not sure that I want anymore of this. Another shock, then another, and another—things are getting serious here. Then like a miracle it is all over, at least for a week when we will be back again. I can dry my feet now and putting my socks and shoes back on, we head off home.

This treatment and a range of many other exercises, some pleasant, some very uncomfortable, meant that over the next few years the strength slowly returned to much of my limbs and I begin to lead a very normal life.

I am seven when my youngest brothers arrive, they are twin boys, and together we make a large family. Poor mum surrounded by five men. At this time we are living in a temporary prefabricated house provided by the council because I was unable to manage the stairs when I got home from hospital and this home had only one floor. It is far too small now that we are six in the family and we move once again to a larger house in Worthing with three bedrooms and a large rear garden backing on to a playing field. In the field we have slides, swings and a roundabout and loads of space for football or chasing.

Mum is not too happy with the location because running down the side of our house is a public footpath that leads to and from the park. Some evenings I can hear things going on in the bushes that apparently I shouldn't be listening to. I don't know what I should be listening for, so am not sure why mum gets in such a fuss. The other night there was a fight on the path, but my brother and I were not allowed to watch. We did hear it though, it sounded great.

When I grow up I want to be an engineer, so today I have decided to build a tunnel from the back of my garden, under the fence and into the park. Getting started is not that hard and I am already about two feet down, but it seems to be getting harder as I get deeper. I am not sure where I can put the stuff that comes out, so I am piling it up behind me.

Right, I think I am deep enough now. If I kneel in the hole, I can just see over the top, so I had better start the tunnel towards the park. As long as I can crawl through, the tunnel will be big enough.

This is tremendous fun. I feel like a prisoner escaping from prison, wait till mum sees this.

I just can't understand why mum and dad are so cross. It was only my first attempt and if dad hadn't stood on the tunnel it wouldn't have collapsed onto me anyway. It is hardly my fault. Early bed with no tea is not the sort of reward a budding young engineer should be getting. I will have to try again later.

Forget tunnelling, go-karting is the sport for me and living on the top of a very steep road, I am surprised that I hadn't thought of it before. Four pram wheels from the local dump, assorted pieces of timber, some string, and my dad's best toolkit and the first prototype go-kart was born. Road testing was not a problem and by the time that I reached the hairpin bend at the bottom of the road I had mastered the controls.

This design, my third, and it has to be said, my best so far, has a sort of roof, two seats and a kind of brake that has yet to be tested. I have decided that this morning would be ideal as mum and dad are in next doors having coffee (they are not happy with the kart being on the road for some reason). What they don't see, they won't worry about, and anyway, my brother Paul owes me a favour.

Getting the kart to the top of the hill is not a problem, now that there are two of us pulling the string and we reach it in no time at all. Both a bit tired but excited by the adventure that lies before us.

I haven't tested the kart carrying two before, (Paul has never been very keen), so I am not sure what difference it will make to the speed, but I always have my new brake. An ideal time to test it out.

Ok, quick push against the kerb, and we're off. Steering with the string is more difficult than I thought. I wish I was using my feet, but there wasn't room with Paul behind me so this will have to do.

We're past our house now—I wish mum and dad could see us, they would be really proud. We are definitely going much faster than I have ever been before.

Right now, let's try the brake. Disappointing, nothing seems to be happening and in fact I don't think it is still attached to the kart. We are about thirty yards from the bend so I will begin pulling on the steering string now...

I was not to know that the string would snap at this point. I haven't had the opportunity to test it under such conditions as this now, and it is really bad luck that the articulated lorry has chosen to come round the bend at the same time that we are, only travelling in the opposite direction. It is my quick thinking in screaming at Paul to duck that enables us to pass completely under the trailer without any harm. I can see the underside of the trailer, the enormous drive shaft spinning around, four pairs of gigantic tyres that look extremely close, and It is only when we meet the concrete kerb on the side of the road that things start to go seriously wrong.

The lorry driver is falling out of his cab and has gone as white as a sheet. He towers above us and had he been calmer would no doubt had said one or two things that perhaps we shouldn't have heard. The rear wheels of his trailer have stopped on top of the kart, we having been thrown onto the pavement by the force of hitting the kerb. Needless to say the kart is not looking it's best, and grasping the opportunity to run, we pick up what remains of the kart and stagger home before mum and dad finds out. I can still hear the driver screaming at us as we throw the damaged vehicle into the shed and rush upstairs. Today is not a good day.

Dad has bought a new motorbike; well it's second-hand, but new to him. A shiny BSA Bantam. Dad is very proud of his motorbike and spends a lot of time cleaning and polishing it in the front garden where he keeps it on a stand. He uses it to get to work.

Today has been a reasonably quiet day, so I have decided to play at being a motorcycle racer and am sitting astride the BSA. It is a really great feeling and I can almost touch the ground with my feet, but not quite. I can hear the crowds roaring and am on the final lap. I can see the chequered flag and stand up to take the cheers and applause. I am not sure why, but my foot has slipped down on to the kick-start and the BSA and I are off. If we hadn't hit the substantial brick wall some six feet in front us which forced us to a sudden stop I could have been seriously hurt. The bike is not really damaged. A bent mudguard, a few broken spokes, and a flat front tyre. I am not certain what happened to the front light, but it was probably my fault. I am not really sure why dad is so angry. I could have been injured.

Somehow I arrive at being ten years old and like most kids of my age am fascinated with cooking. The local electricity company, Seeboard, (I think the company is called) is advertising a 'young chef' competition, and I fancy a go. I am entered into the Southeast heats, and have to prepare and eat, a traditional breakfast for two. By some stroke of good fortune I am now into the various heats finals and my task is to prepare and eat a two-course dinner for two.

I love roast chicken, so this is an ideal choice for me, and I set about preparing the vegetables, meat, etc., and everything goes according to plan. Unluckily I receive a commendation, but not a place in the finals and I am on my way home. I have had a great day, a bit scary, but fun never the less.

We were a very happy family and enjoyed days of endless fun and adventures. We were not by any means well off financially and Dad was always trying to make some extra money for holidays, birthdays, special events, etc.

Today, dad has found himself an old pushcart with large steel and wooden wheels and two long handles to pull or push with.

Dad is going down to the local fruit and vegetable market to buy a selection of items at wholesale prices, and then he and I will be walking around the local streets selling the produce at slightly higher prices.

Dad is ready to go. The cart is laden with produce of all kinds, from tomatoes, peas, beans, cabbages, and potatoes to apples, pears and some rosy red plums, and even some fruits I haven't seen before.

At the top of our road, and then slightly higher still, is a really expensive place to live and dad decides that we will try our luck here. Dragging the cart to the top of the hill is not easy and by the time that we reach the summit and are ready to begin selling we are both tired out.

Initially our efforts are in vain, but very soon some people come out to look at what we have to sale and we begin to progress steadily back down the hill towards home selling a good selection of produce as we go.

Suddenly the front of the cart drops. Dad has let go of the handles, (I think that he thought that I was holding them), and being much lighter than the cart they head very quickly skyward. Gravity takes over once again and the front of the cart hits the road spilling the entire contents on to the carriageway. I am running after apples, oranges, and even potatoes as they speed down the hill.

This is the day that Dad decides that this is not the best way to generate an increase in income, and the idea is scrapped.

I, not unlike many lads of my age, decide that it is time to earn some money for a few of the pleasures of life, so a paper-round is started with the local newsagent. I am pretty good at it. Most of the customers get what they ordered for most of the time, and I always get good tips at Christmas. Some mornings I work in the shop before the papers come in and that is always good fun. I like sorting the papers into rounds and making sure that each round leaves the shop in the correct order of delivery.

This particular morning there is a notice pinned up on the board explaining that there is a national paper boy and girl competition being organised by the Daily Mirror. Mum and Dad have suggested that I have a go so I complete the entry form and send it off. Many of my customers and the newsagent write off in support of my application and incredibly I am sharing the first prize for the Southeast with a papergirl from Eastbourne.

The prize is cash, and a visit to the Royal Banqueting Hall in London as a guest of the

Daily Mirror, and the great day has arrived.

I am dressed in my finest clothes, shoes are gleaming, and mum has checked my hair, and fingernails. I have never been to London on my own before, so I am a bit scared, but now that I am in the taxi taking me to the station, my stomach is beginning to settle.

I am travelling to London by the Brighton Belle (a really posh non-stop London to Brighton train) so have to get to Brighton first. This part of the journey is soon over and I arrive at Brighton station on time to catch my next train.

Walking down the platform that runs beside the train that has recently pulled in from London, I can see that most of the seats are reserved and my heart jumps as I recognise my name printed on a sticker pasted on to one of the windows.

Taking **my** seat I am on my way to London.

I am given refreshments compliments of the Daily Mirror, which is making me feel very important, and too soon we arrive at Victoria.

Victoria station is a vast building with thousands of people rushing about in every direction. So many different types of people, some old, young, small, tall, smart, untidy, even a few tramps. I have never seen so many people together in one place before.

My instructions tell me to make my way towards the taxi rank, which is at the front of the station, so this I do and soon spot a row of taxis waiting for hire. The first one seems available so making my way towards the car, I ask if the driver would take me to the Banqueting Hall. I am soon in the midst of what would appear to be a living stream of vehicles. How we avoid hitting any of them I do not know and it is with great relief that we arrive safely. I pay the fare and make my way up the grand steps towards the open glazed doors.

I am warmly welcomed and guided through a pair of wooden richly ornate panel doors into the finest room that I have ever seen. The whole room is decorated in the warmest and most elegantly coloured wall coverings with brightly shining glass pendant chandeliers reflecting on to a range of beautifully arranged dining tables. Each table is covered in a glorious white cover with each place setting in silver. I am stunned. At the head of the main table is a small stage set up with a microphone and some musical instruments, and seated around me are the other competition winners from across the entire country. I am seated next to the girl from Eastbourne. She seems pleasant enough, but a bit big for me. I am a lot shorter. I must be younger than she is.

The food is lovely and much more than I can manage, although my partner seems to be able to eat it all, and more. I think she is older than I am.

We have an introduction and welcome from the organisers and then the entertainment begins. The first act is a comedian called Dave King. I haven't heard of him, but he is very funny and makes us all laugh. Next, we have a magician called David Nixon who is extremely good and I just can't seem to work out how he does the tricks. When I grow up I would like to do tricks like that. The final act is a group called Cliff Richard and the Shadows and they are brilliant. None of us want them to stop playing or singing, but eventually it is time to leave and we all make our way to our various taxis, trains and then homes. Today has been something special and one day I will look back and smile.

I suppose that I have always had an affinity towards people less fortunate than myself for a number of personal reasons, and one way that a good school friend and I could actually help was to hold regular table top sales from my front garden.

We would collect jumble, books, and collectibles from whomever we could encourage to support our good cause, and by selling them at a tabletop sale on a Saturday morning we would raise a reasonable sum of money. We would then call on the local hospital matron to present our donation for use on the residents and patients. We always enjoyed our visits, which very often included tea and cakes in the matron's study.

Episode 3

Although we all loved our house, we very soon started to grow out of it, and we are transferred to a bigger house nearer to the centre of town.

My school is a fair distance from home so I travel by bicycle, something that I really enjoy although as the years go by it is becoming very exhausting.

I am thirteen when my local GP confirms that a specialist consultant at the Royal National Orthopaedic Hospital, in London should see me.

It will soon be Christmas and mum has promised that after the consultation we will spend some time looking around the many, highly decorated stores that London is so famous for.

Today is the dreaded day and we are to make our way by train. I am anxious this time as before, but for a much different reason. My spine has been twisting around together with my rib cage and this is making my breathing very difficult. The specialist is going to see what can be done to correct it.

One of my teachers at secondary school always picks on one of us during his geography lesson. He is a strange character. None of us actually dislike him. In fact he can be a bit of a joke and is often seen grabbing a chunk of chocolate bar from under his desk when he thinks we aren't looking. He then makes strange burbling noises as he gradually dissolves the chocolate in his mouth. He reminds me of Mr Pickwick in Oliver Dickens.

I seem to be the butt of his comments at the moment and whenever he is near me, he whispers in my ear that unless I sit up straight I will grow deformed. I want to explain that I can't sit up any straighter, but I never get the chance.

Arriving at the London hospital we find the appropriate waiting area, announce our arrival to a very insincere receptionist, and wait. It seems like hours when, suddenly, we are called into a rather dingy consulting room decorated entirely in hospital grey with two rather ornate fluorescent lights hanging from the ceiling by steel links. We are face to face with the specialist consultant.

He looks a serious sort of guy, but with a kind face displaying a friendly smile. A nearby nurse introduces us, explains our reason for attending, and the consultation begins. I am guided down a long winding corridor where I have an endless number of x-rays taken; followed by a series of lung function tests and we are soon back in the waiting area. I am beginning to feel as though I am part of an elaborate experiment and my headaches through the lack of air, and the strange smell that seems to penetrate every part of this building. Hospitals have a peculiar smell that lingers everywhere, constantly reminding you of where you are and what goes on here.

My name is once again called and more than two hours since we first arrived I am back in front of the specialist.

Apparently I have a severe form of spinal scoliosis and unless something is done very soon the situation will become much worse. I don't totally understand what is going on. In fact I don't really care. All I wish for is to get out of this dreadful building and get home.

I gather from the conversation being held with my mum, that I shall have to come into hospital sometime early next year and it could be a long stay. Things do not look too good.

We look around many of the shops and try to forget the earlier events, for a while, at least and are soon heading back home.

Christmas comes and goes and soon after my fourteenth birthday, the dreaded day arrives.

I have to report to the Royal National Orthopaedic Hospital in Stanmore, Middlesex, and mum and dad drive me there in dad's car.

On arrival I am taken to see the Staff Nurse who shows me where my bed is and where I can change my clothes, etc. This has to be the most frightening day of my life. The ward is like an army barracks with very high ceilings, lights suspended from the ceiling, long stretches of tall windows, and that smell. Spaced on all sides and down the centre of the ward are young kids like me, in all forms of plaster casts. Some have got arms and legs hanging by wires and pulleys and look very uncomfortable. The guy in the bed next to mine is covered in plaster from his neck to his waist and yet seems remarkably happy. Perhaps he is going home soon.

It is time to say goodbye to mum and dad and I feel awful. I know I am going to cry— I can feel it building up inside me and it is going to boil over. I don't want them to leave me here. It's terrible. It's frightening.

They have gone. I am absolutely alone, miles from home and no one to talk to. I can only run into the toilets down the corridor and cry my heart out. What happens to me if they crash on the way home? Nobody will know that I am here? I might not see mum and dad ever again. Why am I here? I want to hold mum and dad as tightly as I can. I didn't say goodbye properly.

I am guided by a nurse back to my bed, told to change into a special gown and wear some appalling sort of thong, and wait for the doctor to visit. I am embarrassed, scared, alone, in fact over the next few hours I go through every conceivable negative feeling.

My surgeon is very friendly and tries to put me at ease. Mum and dad will be up to see me at the weekend (that's nearly five days away), and I have lots of tests to go through. The first one is tomorrow morning and the nurse will be with me all of the time. Now I can have a meal, watch some television, and try to get to know my companions. I just can't forget mum and dad. I want to see them. I want to see my brothers. I want to go home. The tears well up again and I can't stop myself from crying. I don't want anything to eat. I don't want to watch television. I just want to go home. I am not ill. I can run and walk and play and jump as good as any of my friends, so why am I in this dreadful place. This is not fair.

Last night I cried my self to sleep and am woken by one of the many nurses telling me that it was time to have a wash ready for breakfast. Apparently it will be brought to me on a tray, but I can take it to the table at the end of the ward if I would like to. Curtains are being drawn and I can see out into the gardens that surround the ward. Actually in the morning light it looks quite pleasant, and I can see loads of small birds scrabbling around on the grass for the early worm.

Breakfast is scrambled egg (which I quite like), and toast and jam, and we can have tea or orange juice. I said that I didn't really want orange, so was given a small mug of hot, sweet tea.

Nurses (or orderlies as I found out later) are already polishing the floor and screens surround some of the beds. I found out to my horror what was going on behind these screens a few days later.

Breakfast is soon over and nurses visit us all. My nurse takes my temperature and pulse, and then asks me if I have emptied my bowels today. I hadn't, and this was noted on a chart that was attached to my bed.

It is now nine o'clock, and I am taken through the rubber doors at one end of the ward and into a small laboratory type area. The walls are littered with instruments and equipment that don't look as though they have been used for years, and glancing at some of them, I hope they never are.

I am told to stand on a small wooden box with my back to the wall and my height is measured. From this moment on, and for what feels like the entire morning, I am subjected to a myriad of different tests and experiments until eventually I am told that it is time for lunch.

To be honest, the food in the hospital wasn't bad. It was very similar to that at school, but with larger portions and more variety, although for the first few days I ate very little.

Three o'clock and it is visiting time and the fear and misery returns. I have no visitors. As far as I can tell every other patient has at least one visitor, their mum or dad, or perhaps an aunt or uncle. They have books, magazines, fruit, bottles of drink and more importantly a hug. The torment continues for at least an hour. The visitors are given tea and biscuits, and I can hear laughter and chatter filling the ward. I feel really desperate. I have read my magazines. I can't watch the television as it is at the other end of the ward, and

I feel sick. I gather that there is another session for visitors in the evening.

I have a visit from my surgeon who is reading my notes and discussing the next moves with the staff nurse at the foot of my bed. "Well Peter", he says, smiling, "On Friday you are going to get fitted for the first plaster cast. It won't hurt, in fact some patients actually find it fun". I bet they do.

I sleep better tonight and am beginning to reconcile myself to being here. It won't be for long, hopefully, and I can be back home again.

"Have you emptied your bowels today?" I am going through the now familiar early morning get you up routine and finding the question less embarrassing. I answer in the affirmative and this pleases my nurse. I shall have to go soon, but I just don't seem to be able to at the moment.

The walk to the plaster area is quite long and I am being taken by a friendly Indian porter who knows his way around the hospital like the back of his hand. He is telling me all sorts of stories about what he has seen. I am not certain about a few of them.

We have arrived and I am asked to remove my top and lie down on the long trolley parked in the centre of the room. The trolley is covered with a maroon coloured rubber mat and is cold to the touch. There are two nurses in here, and a guy who looks like a doctor, but I am not sure if he is or not. I am given a sort of string vest to wear and layer by layer the 'doctor' is wrapping me with strips of wet, cold, plaster. One of the nurses holds my head back and the plaster is taken up under my chin and around the back of my neck. The cast sets very quickly and I feel trapped in a plaster straitjacket with holes for my arms to poke through. There is a small gap that stretches around just under my ribs, and then a further cast that extends down to my hipbone. I can move nothing above my hip except for my arms, sticking out each side like a tailor's dummy.

I am taken back to the ward on the trolley and deposited unceremoniously onto my bed where I lie absolutely demoralised.

I am shortly to discover what goes on behind the screens, as I ask a nurse if I could use the toilet. My bowels need emptying now! How degraded I feel. This is the first time that I ever remember seeing a bedpan, and to have to ask a nurse for assistance I felt completely embarrassed. If only I had known this before, I would have tried much harder before the plaster episode. The smell seems to hang around and I know that everyone in the ward knows what I am doing. I am as red as a beetroot, covered in balls of sweat and wish that I could die, NOW.

The situation seems to be getting worse and worse, surely it can't continue?

Saturday, and apparently it can. I am fitted with two long steel bolts that connect both halves of the cast and run down each side of my torso. The bolts are plastered onto the cast and the whole assembly becomes extremely rigid.

Sunday, and joy of joys, mum and dad have arrived. This is wonderful. They have not changed a bit. Mum looks a bit tired, but very happy to see me and I cannot explain the joy of seeing them again. I have new magazines, some fruit, drink, and letters and cards from many friends and relations. Even my brothers have sent a present. They are staying with nanny while mum and dad visits. Visiting time is over far too soon and promising to telephone me when they get home, mum and dad leave. I can do nothing but wave them goodbye and sink into a feeling of gloom once again.

It is ages since they left and still no phone call. Perhaps they had a crash. Maybe they are ill, or injured. What can I do trapped in this plaster cast? "Peter, your mum telephoned and they send their love" a nurse passes on the message and the world is slightly brighter.

Yesterday, whilst mum and dad were here, the surgeon had explained the process of straightening my spine and it is to start today. Over the next few weeks, the bolts on my cast will be extended a little more each day, until I have been stretched sufficiently to remove some of the curvature from my spine. Once this has been achieved, I will have an operation to graft bone tissue around my spine to support it in this new position. The operation is known as a spinal fusion and is generally very successful.

This afternoon I have had the bolts extended and I feel taller already. The pressure on my chin is rather an odd sensation, although my ribs and hip take most of the force. I am finding it very difficult to eat, or drink, and prefer using a straw.

I am permitted to get up and walk around the ward, in fact, this is encouraged, but I am finding it a very uncomfortable experience. The bottom of the cast tends to rub on my hip when I walk, and I am already developing a sore.

Sleeping is exceptionally uncomfortable, and I have to turn over as one solid mass using a sort of throwing movement. The bed clothes get caught on the bolts and usually I end up with nothing on top of me which is both highly embarrassing, and somewhat annoying as I have to keep asking one of the night nurses if they could replace them for me. I haven't yet got to use a 'bottle', but I am sure that this 'pleasure' will come.

Last Sunday's visit was a real nightmare for my poor parents. Apparently, some thirty miles from home, their car had broken down and ground to a halt on a lonely road not usually carrying much traffic. The weather, typically, was appalling with sheets of water covering the road and a cold Northerly wind blowing leaves and small objects high into the overcast star-less night sky.

They had waited in desperation for almost an hour, when a local farmer drove up in his tractor to enquire if there was anything that he could do to help. Within the hour my parents were being towed home, attached to the tractor by a steel bar through which they felt every bump and judder from the tractor. It was two hours later that they finally reached home, gave the farmer something for his extremely kind act, and retired exhausted to bed.

This coming Sunday, we are all to be told what is to happen next and going by my past experiences I am not going to like what I hear.

Well, now I have heard everything. My operation is planned for next Tuesday; it is a lengthy and complicated process and will last for at least eight hours. Mum is going to stay over night in a parent's accommodation block next door. Following the operation, I have to stay in bed, horizontal, encased in a full cast of plaster for six months. Six months. This is half an entire year. Surely this can't be right. Evidently it is.

Tuesday morning and I am back in the world of fear and trepidation. I am not allowed to have anything to eat or drink and I have been given a rather weird pill, which is deposited in a most unusual part of my body. The effects are almost immediate and very unpleasant.

I am now on my way to the plaster room where I am to have the cast removed and replaced by a temporary steel brace known as a 'Milwaukee'. The 'doctor' is wielding an electric rotary saw and I feel that I am about to be dismembered. Grinding into the side of my cast alongside one of the bolts, great clouds of plaster dust is thrown into the air and my immediate thought is how does the 'doctor' know when he has cut through the plaster and reached me. I am dreading the fact that I may find out before he does. I think he has noticed the extreme look of panic on my face, as he lifts the saw from my cast and moves it towards his own arm. Immediately the blade touches his jacket, the saw stops. I am so relieved, that I do not notice that the cast has now been removed and is being replaced by the new 'skeleton' brace that will hold my spine in place throughout the operation.

Wheeled back to the ward I am confused with a combination of fear and some relief.

Mum has arrived and looks as concerned as I feel. She is giving me a hug when I receive the 'premed' injection and I am all set.

An hour or so has passed. A shiny new trolley arrives pushed by a smart looking nurse, and I am gently lifted on to it, say goodbye to mum and disappear through the rubber doors.

I can see a range of brightly-lit lights; shiny steel instruments, highly polished floors, and two or three doctors dressed in white gowns and caps. One of them approaches me and I can see that he is holding a syringe. "Peter, when I ask you, would you please start counting down from ten, and you will fall fast asleep" With that strange smell filling my nose, Ten, Nine, Eight...
Focusing is a little difficult, and trying to determine what I am doing here, wherever here is, is a real challenge. I can hear voices, and through the mist I think that I can make out some people wandering about. My back is unimaginably sore, and for some inexplicable reason my hips hurt too. My mouth and throat feel like they are on

fire, and I would die for a drink. My head aches like it has never ached before and..

I haven't moved, but I can see one or two objects a bit clearer now that the mist has started to clear. It's just like looking through a dirty window. I know that I am lying on my back and I can move my arms but not a lot else.

I can sense that there is someone beside me, but to move to have a look really hurts, so I will give that a miss. I have a tube filled with clear liquid going into my left arm, and one with red liquid (probably blood) going into the other. I have just realised that mum is sitting beside the bed, but I don't think she has noticed that I am awake yet. My back feels as though I have been sliced with a 'Stanley' knife, it is excruciatingly painful and whenever I move I have a sensation of tearing something.

Mum has spotted me looking and is holding my hand. It feels lovely and I can see a smile forming across her face. A doctor has come into the room and is talking to mum. I am being given a small injection in my arm and soon fall asleep once more.

The operation would (at least initially), appear to have been successful. It had taken just over eight hours and I have been given eight pints of blood since the operation began. The main concern now is that I recover my strength as soon as possible so that I can be returned to the ward. I have never had a major operation before and I am experiencing a whole range of sensations, from being in complete control to frightening hallucinations, and all stages between.

As insignificant as it appears today, over forty years later, the only really solid event that I can remember whilst I was going through this period of recovery, was when I accidentally discovered that if I clenched my fist, I could send streams of bubbles up the two tubes. As my focus improved I would send the bubbles to the top declaring one of the tubes as winner.

Mum is fantastic and soon I am asking all sorts of questions concerning the operation and what happens next. It is within a couple of days, that I am transferred back to the ward and my own bed. The nurses are looking after me magnificently and constantly check my scars, take my temperature, pulse, and blood for testing. I am receiving two injections a day, one in the morning, the other late afternoon, and with the exception of the soreness from the two scars I begin to feel better everyday.

Mum went home on Thursday with the promise that she and dad would return Sunday, and this I was really looking forward to.

Ten days have passed since the day of the operation. Sunday certainly did see the return of mum and dad, which was wonderful, and I am having my stitches removed later this morning. I have fifty-four of them down my back, and eighteen on my hip, where the bone was taken to graft on to my spine. A nurse is soon here and I am gently rolled on to my front. I feel every one of the seventy-two stitches being removed with almost every one producing tears in my eyes. Some of them have been pulled too tight, and the skin has started to grow over the stitch. These beauties have to be pulled through the scar tissue. The scars are dressed with a soft, warm smelling fabric and I am gently rolled back over. The soreness has certainly begun to ebb and I am feeling a lot more comfortable.

Once the doctors are satisfied that the scar tissue is healing correctly, I am refitted with the plaster cast (this time in one piece stretching from my chin to my hip) and reminded not to try to sit up or move around inside the cast.

Today I am off to the hospital dentist. Apparently the cast under my chin may be pushing my front top teeth out of line (I have never understood this and am convinced it is a confidence trick to get me to the dentist). Some people have the knack of being able to judge a person by the first impression, but a three-year-old child could judge this particular character with not a bad thought in his head. The dentist looked as though he hated his job, his patients, in fact life, and did all he could to express these feelings in the treatment of the poor longsuffering children that he was supposed to help.

I am wheeled by trolley into the surgery and told to lie still (If I could have done anything else—I would have been extremely surprised). The dentist, muttering under his foul smelling breath (no masks in these days) places a small steel banana shaped container into my mouth and I am asked to clench my teeth together. Biting into a warm mass of molten plastic material is not what I had expected and I immediately panic that I may not get my teeth apart anymore, or if I do, several of them will be left in the plastic goo.

"Open wide" and he withdraws the container as you would scoop out an oyster from its shell.

This again is not a good day. It is not so much about what is going on, more about the feeling of complete helplessness trapped in a plaster coffin on a steel and rubber trolley miles from home and civilisation. Here I have no control over what is going on, my questions and concerns go completely unheeded and I have no one to turn to.

Five days later and it is time to have the brace fitted. The same miserable dentist is here and holding my face with one hand, he eases the brace on to my top teeth. It is rubbing on my gum, which starts to bleed. The brace is removed, filed with a tool that looks as though it was used during the Civil war as a weapon of torture, and refitted. Apparently one of the teeth sections is slightly out of line, so the offending tooth is removed. He has just taken my tooth out! No gas, no painkiller, no warning, Nothing. At this precise moment one of my teeth is trapped in the end of a malicious pair of forceps. I can not believe what has just happened. What has this barbaric man done to me? Without pausing for a breath, the brace is re-fitted, and I am wheeled back to the ward. Definitely not a good day.

Now when I eat, I not only have to try and enjoy my meal lying on my back, Or if I ask a nurse, on my side, I have also to suck the food, and prevent it going up and behind the brace which fits snugly into the roof of my mouth. I have had enough of this. I cannot take any more and the brace is removed and hidden under my pillow. I am now going to spend the next six months worrying about the condition and shape of my front teeth. I might not look like the Hunchback of Notre-Dame, but probably Bugs Bunny.

One of my favourite television programmes at the moment is 'Emergency Ward 10'. Goodness knows why, but is does cheer me up. This evening it begins at seven o'clock, and somehow I have to arrange my bed so that I can see, and just as importantly, hear it. I am currently at the far end of the ward, furthest from the screen. I have become friends with a number of kids in here, with one of them having his leg stretch. Apparently it is three inches shorter than his other leg because of a hip problem. He has taught me how to drag my bed up the ward by pulling on each bed as I go by until I get close enough to the screen. Regrettably the beds have wheel locks to prevent just this kind of manoeuvring so my first task is to find someone to unlock my wheels.

One of the lads across the way is in for a foot operation and is still relatively mobile. It takes very little persuasion for him to release the locks. Pulling on the beds is a bit of a strain and occasionally I can feel the scars twitching, but eventually I roll into position and the programme begins. The staff nurse is never very impressed by this tactical move, but as the other nurses on our ward are part of the night shift, they don't really seem to mind. I think it must be quite boring working through the night, after all, we aren't ill, so rarely need anything, except for the dreaded bed-pan of course.

This particular evening the programme is showing one of the doctors playing with a small game in which he has to roll a tiny ball along a series of alley ways, (avoiding many pit holes) to arrive at the finishing post. It looks very difficult but enormous fun. I shall have to try to get one of those.

A week later, a small package is delivered to my bed, and with rising excitement I tear open the wrapping to discover the very game being played on the television last week. Inside the wrapping, a letter from one of the actors, Desmond Carrington, explains that he is very pleased to receive my note enquiring about the game. He goes on to say that the actual game is one of the studio's props and can't be forwarded, so instead he has bought a similar one in the hope that I will enjoy it whilst I am in hospital. I just can't believe it and will cherish his letter for a long time.

Visiting times in the ward are not so depressing now as I am getting a few regular visits from some very kind people that mum and dad met in a shop up here one Sunday. The family has two daughters about my age and they often call in with time for a chat, a laugh, and the latest comics that I read and pass around the ward. Even my old great aunt living in Walthamstowe calls in occasionally during the week, which is a great treat.

I have been at Stanmore now for almost two months and although I am starting to see the nurses, doctors, and fellow patients as one big family, I still want to go home. I have my GCE examinations in just over a year and need to get good grades, as I want to go into the Customs and Excise Department, or Air Traffic Control. We do have a teacher who comes in every day with work to do, or to talk through a particular subject, but it is not like being at school.

Mum and dad have been having discussions with the doctors about me being allowed to go home, with perhaps a health visitor calling in me once a day. Eventually, agreement is reached and I am prepared for the journey home.

Saying goodbye to my friends at Stanmore is much more difficult than I anticipated, but I am soon loaded into an ambulance and on my way home. Yes!

Episode 4

My homecoming is a cauldron of emotions. I am happy, sad, tearful, frightened, worried, and excited all at the same time. The butterflies in my stomach have decided to escape through my throat, and my heart thinks that I have just completed a three-minute mile.

I am gently lifted from the ambulance by stretcher and carried carefully into our living room. Mum has set my bed by the window and I can see into our garden. The view is wonderful, the smell is home, and I am exceedingly happy.

The plan is that I am to stay here for four months, laying horizontally, encased in the plaster jacket, until it is time for me to return to Stanmore to have the cast removed. I shall be having a teacher call every morning to help me with my studies and a health visitor will also call in case mum or I have any concerns.

It is great to be part of our family again and I am soon back in amongst the gossip and experiences of my three younger brothers who help me in every way possible. Dad is much relieved at not having to travel to Stanmore every Sunday. I think it has really worn him out, although he never shows it.

I am still having to use the dreaded bedpan and of course now I am home mum has to help me. I don't know how she manages it all, with me an added bother to her already busy life looking after dad and my three brothers.

I am going out for a walk today. Mum and dad have managed to get hold of a trolley from the local hospital that we can borrow, so that I can be taken around the town for a spot of fresh air and a change of scenery. It has just been delivered and I am devastated. It looks exactly like a wooden coffin, but on wheels. It has four quite high sides, a base, and handles along each side. Laying in it, I cannot quite see over the top and feel highly embarrassed. "How is Peter today?"

"Doesn't Peter look well", "Is he enjoying his trip out?" Hold on, I'm not deaf, or daft. I _can_ talk, why don't you try talking to me. I am on display, part of a macabre exhibition, being transported around the town for people to look at and wonder. "Oh poor boy", "How did he end up like that?"

I am not enjoying this at all. I am annoyed and embarrassed, and want to go home. Why are people so hurtful and tactless?

The last four months have passed very quickly and the transport has arrived for the return journey to Stanmore. Gently transported into the ambulance, we are soon off and heading for the ward once more.

Nothing much has changed, there are several new patients, and many of my old friends have been discharged and gone home. I recognise some of the nurses, who seem very tall. I hadn't noticed this before; how strange.

Today is the big day and I am off to have the plaster cast removed. I shall miss it after all this time and it is covered with signatures collected over the last six months. I am transported to the plaster room and using the very same saw as before, I am released. What a strange feeling, and the smell of dried skin, dirt and goodness knows what else. A bed bath is in order and I thoroughly relish the experience. Wonderful.

I can move about on my bed, but I must not get up until the Milwaukee brace has been fitted which will be tomorrow. I can't explain the joy of being able to lie in bed and actually feel the covers. I am a bit worried about my back, which doesn't appear to be as straight as I thought it would be. However the doctors assure me that it is.

The brace is fitted and I sit up for the first time for six months. Incredible, everything is so much smaller than I thought. It is a long way to the floor and swinging my legs over the side of the bed, I am not certain that they won't reach the floor. But they do. Walking, however, is another thing altogether and I have completely forgotten how to do it.

It has taken me almost a week of exercise and parallel bars while towering over the nurses (who are surprisingly short) to learn how to walk again and I am still not very confident. One of the hip supports has been rubbing on my hip and has produced a sore that is proving difficult to heal. I am not going to be let home until this clears, and it is not looking very promising.

Seven days later, the sore has healed sufficiently for me to be discharged from hospital and I am to be allowed home tomorrow. This is excellent news and I am overjoyed.

I feel very important, I have an ambulance that is taking me to Victoria Station, and it drives right on to the platform, parking alongside the train that has a carriage reserved for just for mum and I.

Back home and other than the restrictions of the brace, I am trying to get back to normal. I can actually use the toilet properly now so that is a relief, and feel much more independent.

I am having a home teacher for a couple of weeks and then following a check-up with my doctor I can return to school. I am considerably apprehensive about going to school. Not the physical part, but the response that I might get from my schoolmates and those who don't know me. Teenagers can be very harsh and don't always consider what they are saying.

Return to school was great. None of my fears materialised and everyone took me back as though I had never been away. The only negative response was from some of the younger guys who complained that I had a taxi to take me to and from school, and they had to walk.

For six months I wore the brace. I could take it off at night, and towards the end, some parts of the day but I was glad when the day came for me to return to London to have my final check-up.

It was confirmed that I could have the brace removed permanently as long as I was careful for the next few weeks and had regular checks with my GP in Worthing. The bad news was that the operation had not been as successful as they had hoped. I would continue to have a protruding shoulder blade and some rib cage displacement, which although would not get any worse could be disfiguring. I had two alternatives; I could undertake the whole operation again and spend the next 6 months back at Stanmore, or; a plastic surgeon would remove my shoulder blade which would cause my right arm to be useless. I took the third alternative, said no thanks, and returned home with mum.

It is a peculiar situation because before I went though the past twelve months I had not bothered about my appearance at all. Now I am very conscious of my deformity, and feel that I have been cheated out of a year of my life. I understand that without the operation my breathing would have become very restricted as the curve of my spine and rib cage increased. I would not be able to do the things that I can now do, but my appearance is very important to me at fifteen years of age and I feel let down.

I am certain that people with whom I meet notice my curvature. They will not mention it, but I can see them glancing at my back and stomach as we talk. Regrettably, the plaster cast worn for six months whilst I was still growing has also seriously affected the development of my chest, and has left me barrel-chested. I am not disabled in the real sense of the word. I can do everything that any teenager can do. Maybe not so well, or for so long, but I can participate, and I do. I must lead a normal life and get as much out of it as I can. In some respects I would like my disability to be more obvious, maybe use a stick, or limp, and then people wouldn't expect quite so much.

During the summer holidays I have a job working in an ice-cream kiosk directly on the beach. My speciality is 'frothy coffee', ice-cream whips with a chocolate stick, and the traditional candyfloss. This is great fun and I am making loads of new friends. The pay is not too good, but to a hot-blooded teenage boy, the opportunity to serve ice-cream and candy-floss to hundreds of delicious bikini clad girls, is pay enough.

My GCE examinations come and go, and I obtain some reasonable grades. I am not accepted into the Customs and Excise through failure of their medical, and I change my mind about the Air Traffic Control after reading about the enormous stress that many of the teams go through. I spend some time at the local Sixth Form College working for three A Levels, but decide that earning some real money is more important, and begin training as a Quantity Surveyor with a local practice.

I am determined that my physical condition will not stop me from participating in normal activities so on my seventeenth birthday and very first holiday without the rest of the family, I take a ten day coach holiday to Austria. Picking up the coach from Victoria Coach Station we are very soon heading through France. The coach has two drivers to permit the coach to be driven non-stop and as we are speeding along one of the Autobahns, the present driver locks the steering wheel, leaves his seat and is strolling casually to the rear of the coach meeting his colleague coming forward. Just as casually, the new driver sits in the seat, unlocks the wheel and continues the journey.

Toilet stops are sparse and after 8 hours sitting on a bouncy coach seat trying to get some sleep, desperation begins to set in. There are no toilet facilities on the coach, and the next stop we are informed is 80 miles away. I calculate this to be about two hours. (I have always been good at arithmetic—I achieved a GCE grade 1). This doesn't help however, as I doubt that I will last that long. I do manage to last. I cross my legs as hard as I can. I think about anything other than liquids and even try to sleep, but succeed I do, and the relief I feel as we pull into the service area is immeasurable.

Austria is marvellous and prides itself on one of the highest publicly accessible mountains in Europe. One of the programmed tours is to the very top of this mountain and having been told in London that I should avoid extreme heights due to a thinning of the air and a shortage of oxygen, the challenge was accepted.

It is beautiful up here, I can see for miles and miles. Across the white capped peaks of many smaller mountains covered in pine trees and maroon heather, down into distant valleys where thin snakes of blue are winding their way through forests of every shade of green, and where I feel that I can almost touch the icy blue sky. The air is crisp and still. I am standing on about two foot of freshly compressed snow and I can hear the soft crunching sound as I slowly walk around the fenced summit. My steps are easy. I feel light and free. My breathing is short and difficult, but the complete awe of what I behold is worth every moment. I feel that I am a tiny part of some enormous plan, a character in a well-written play with the scenery painted by someone inspired. I feel good.

Austria is a country that I shall return to again, and one day, maybe, bring a friend.

My first very own vehicle is a Triumph motorcycle and I have months of good honest fun touring the local highways and byways and gradually I work my way through a selection of models including a motorcycle and sidecar combination.

The local Volunteer Emergency Service (VES) is recruiting new members and I join up. My duties are to support the various emergency services by transporting equipment and supplies to area in need and where alternative sources of transport are either not available or not suitable.

One of my first jobs is to transport a few pints of blood from our local hospital to a clinic in Horsham and from here on in, I am called to assist at least two or three times a week. The service is very rewarding and there is a feeling of great comradeship amongst the members.

The last motorcycle that I had the pleasure of owning was a small 'Honda 50'. A nippy little bike with not a lot of power, but a comfortable bike to ride and the unusual luxury of an electric starter.

My brother and I travelled around quite a lot on the Honda, and this morning we have decided to visit Gatwick Airport for a spot of plane watching. I have had some problems with the bike in that it seems to be loosing oil, but my local workshop have cured the leak so this will be like a road test.

We are travelling at about forty miles an hour down the long A23 into Crawley. The road is reasonably quiet, except for one or two vehicles behind us; one of which as I am to discover later is a police car. Forty miles per hour is a comfortable speed for the Honda, especially carrying a passenger, so as we begin to gather speed down the hill, I decide to gently apply the brakes. The next few hours have been completely wiped from my memory, but this is what happened according to the following police car.

On applying the brakes, the rear wheel locked and skidded on a patch of oil that had been dripping on to the tyre ever since we left Worthing. The bike had swerved to the left, and struck the kerb, throwing me over the handlebars and depositing my passenger untidily onto the road landing on his bottom. According to the policeman, he had called the ambulance even before I struck my head, splitting open my crash helmet, on the road verge.

Transportation to hospital is still a blur, and I can only remember waking up in the accident ward almost six hours later suffering from concussion and a slight fracture. My brother had several bruises that prevented him from sitting down for quite a few days. As for the flying through the air—I can remember nothing at all.

Eventually I manage to afford to purchase a car and am the proud owner of a second-hand black Ford Consul. I am officially appointed as my groups of friends' locals free taxis and spend a fortune shuttling them around Worthing and West Sussex.

It is Saturday afternoon and five friends and I have just left a stockcar race meeting held at a large track near Eastbourne, some twenty miles from home. It has been raining steadily all day, which to be honest, has enhanced the track events considerably, and the roads are flooded as we head down a long hill to meet a swollen ford at the bottom. Travelling at speed the spray from each wheel is very impressive as we hit the water and we are soon speeding away up the hill on the other side. Reaching the brow of the hill, the car once again is heading down hill and I notice that ahead of us there is a sharp bend to the left. Nearing the bend I apply the brakes.. Nothing happens, I might just as well be dragging my feet. Instead of braking we actual speed up as we approach the bend.

I have two choices; I can either warn my friends (who are completely oblivious to what is about to occur), or; keep quiet and hope that I make the bend. I decide to do neither as I could see that there wasn't any way that we would make the bend at this speed. Through the hedge directly on the bend and ahead of me appeared to be some sort of gate. Whether it was open or not, I could not make out, but it had to be better than trying to round the bend.

It is quite a few seconds before my friends realise that something is wrong and by now we are shaking our way down an old farm track slowly grinding to a halt almost one hundred yards from the road. The gate had been open. The brakes dry out in about thirty minutes and we resume out journey home.

Over the next couple of years I owned a Triumph herald, a Ford Cortina Mk 1, and an ex Army Armoured Car. I am not certain why I bought this, probably on a whim, but it could go underwater, so this was possibly the thought in mind.

Whilst going through these adventures I was still living at home, and dad often kept a few chickens in the rear garden. The eggs were delicious and as the chickens ceased laying they were killed and either cooked, or if they were too old, buried or disposed of in the dustbin.

This particular morning dad has decided to slaughter a couple of the older hens and as they are far too old to eat proposes to dispose of them in the usual manner. Dad, however, was very concerned that none of his hens should suffer any pain or discomfort. One of his hens recently had been particularly difficult to slaughter by the traditional method of wringing its neck, and so had decided to behead them instead. At least this is quick and positive, if not quite the recognised method to be adopted when slaughtering chickens.

Holding the first chicken firmly down on the chopping block, dad brings down the axe with a firm swing beheading the chicken immediately with one strike. Dad picks up the dead hen and drops it into the plastic bag lining the bin. It is possibly ten or so seconds later, when with a ghostly rustle of feathers, the headless chicken appears from inside the bin and begins to throw itself around the garden. I know that in some cases the nerve endings of some chickens can still react quite a few seconds after death, but all of our chickens died of natural causes from this day onwards.

Dad had many different jobs whilst my brothers and I were growing up and was well known and respected up to and after his death almost 20 years ago. One of the highlights of his life, for me, was when he opened his own second hand furniture and haulage business in a fairly large 'lock-up' shop near the centre of town. I spent very many happy weekends working with dad in the shop, and quite often assisted with household removals and haulage contracts.

This particular Saturday morning comes to mind when dad asks me if I would collect a small piano from an address about ten miles away and deliver it to a piano shop in the town. Taking the company van, I pick up my cousin (who has volunteered to help), and head towards the pick-up address. Apparently the piano is a 'baby grand' and will be little problem to us young lads. The 'baby' is a standard grand piano currently located in the front room of a very small basement flat.

The access to the flat is down a set of winding steel staircase treads and through a door that a traditional piano would have sneered at. The only other access was through a very tired looking vertical timber sash window of which only the top half appeared to open. Attempting to lift the piano, I managed to clear about six inches from the floor, which was not a lot of good when we had to move it almost 20 feet to the van and almost 12 feet vertically. A problem is only a challenge waiting to be solved. An impossible task is to move this piano.

I am reliably informed that the legs of the piano can be removed, This will make it easier to handle, but has absolutely no effect on the weight. I resolve that the only we are going to get the piano into the van is to 'bribe' a few passers by. After almost thirty minutes I have rounded up four able looking guys (at considerable cost) and we begin the move. I have taken out both sashes of the window (the owner assures me that she will be able to replace them, although to be honest, I have my sincere doubts that that will ever be possible again), and the piano is eventually manhandled on to the floor of the van.

We have about thirty minutes of travelling time to remove some of the 'minor' scratches and securing the piano with our strongest webbing I begin the journey homeward. My partner agreed to stand in the back of the van with the piano (well it is my dads van), to check its stability en-route. All is well, just ten minutes to go, most of the scratches have been removed, and it hasn't been too bad after all. Rounding a slight bend, I notice a young lad about to step on to the road. I don't think I stopped particularly sharply, and I did shout a warning, but there was a loud snapping sound, which resounded around the van, and the piano and my cousin entered the drivers cab.

I am not convinced that the owner of the piano shop where we eventually deliver the piano, knows why we are grinning as we pull up outside his shop, but they quickly disappeared when he informs us that he presently alone, and has a hernia.

Dad assured us that he had been told it was a 'baby grand' and on the ground floor, but I have always wondered why he didn't do that particular delivery.

This weekend, having just achieved my Heavy Goods Vehicle driving licence (HGV - Class 1), I have been asked to deliver a number of 'flat-pack' kitchen units to a small town in Wales and am looking forward to the trip immensely. I am driving a large high-sided box unit lorry.

The journey so far has been very uneventful, and I am soon driving into the extremely picturesque town of Ross-On-Wye in South Wales. One of the main streets is quite steep and with queues of traffic behind and in front of me I am crawling up the hill to a set of traffic lights on the brow. The lights change to red and we all screech to a halt. The sounds of my air brakes hissing like an old steam train coming to rest. Red and Amber, Green, I am off. Well, not quite. Everything has gone dead. I have no power at all, the engine has died on me leaving me without any electrical supply, brakes, or steering. The only thing stopping me from rolling down hill and into the cars waiting patiently behind me is the emergency hand brake, which I lock on. I very rarely panic, but I am in a situation that I have no idea how to resolve. There is a tap on the passenger door and a smart gentleman introducing himself as the local traffic warden asks if I have a problem. I carefully go through the various options with him and together we decide that the only thing that I can do is to slowly! reverse down the hill and into a parking area some one hundred yards behind me.

Using the emergency brake in a series of short on/off movements I reverse the lorry down the hill through a clearing in the traffic formed by the traffic warden, and gradually come to halt in the parking area. Needless to say, I am annoyed, exhausted and covered in beads of perspiration. Jumping down from the cab, I slam the driver's door shut, to, to my complete amazement and disbelief, suddenly hear the sound of my hazard warning lights flashing nonchalantly away as though nothing is wrong. Every part of the system is back on and working. I very quickly make the delivery and head back home.

As my brothers and I grew older we would very often help during our holidays or at weekends with the occasional house removal, and this particular morning dad has asked if we would help him with a complete house clearance. The owners have split up and are selling their unwanted property. Dad has borrowed the key from a neighbour and we arrive outside the small terraced house in town. Our initial reaction upon entering the property is one of surprise as there are no signs of packing; in fact the rooms look 'lived in'. We have, however, met all sorts of client in the past and so begin the process of packing, boxing, and transferring to the lorry.

Many of the items are not suitable for re-sale so these we pack in separate containers for disposal at the local 'tip', with the remainder being transferred to our shop for valuation and purchase. The day has gone smoothly, all of the items have been dispatched to their appropriate destinations and a cheque is made out to the owners for the objects purchased. Entering the shop are two quite smart looking men, holding identification cards. They are from the local police station and are detectives looking into the illegal removal of property from a house in town. It would seem that a neighbour had spotted several men transferring goods from the house into a lorry. The description given of the lorry fitted dads perfectly.

It is an odd sort of day, starting well, developing smoothly and now it seems we are to be charged with theft. We have been taken for a ride by a rather upset husband who, when his wife admits to having an affair, arranges for a local furniture company to enter his wife's house and remove her belongings while she is away on holiday. We haven't been charged with any offence, dad has lost a fair bit of money (the goods have to be returned), and I decide that the removal business is not for me.

Three weeks later and dad has been offered an unusual job to transport a lorry load of furniture and belongings to a newly built flat in Northern France. I have taken the lorry over to France on a couple of occasions but not an entire lorry full. Naturally, and without thinking, I agree to drive the large furniture lorry and early this morning we are on our way to Dover to catch the mid morning ferry to Calais.

Customs and Excise at Dover check the mountain of paperwork that we have to complete and I am then instructed to board the ferry. On this particular ferry we are asked to reverse the vehicle in to place and normally this would not be a problem but my comprehension of the French language at this time is suspect. The ferrymen could only speak French (or so it seemed). Almost causing an international incident our lorry is eventually parked where 'they' want it and we mount the stairway for much needed refreshments. All to soon, the port of Calais is reached and we are disembarked into the incoming goods area where our manifest is checked.

I think the biggest mistake that we made was to be too honest as we had listed every piece of furniture that we were carrying, from the dining room table to a nondescript little picture taken from the guest bathroom. "Picture, monsieur ", I am approached by a small French gentleman, pointing to item number 45; picture, entered on the paperwork. I explain that it is a very small print of a flock of geese flying across a lake, and in any case it was one of the first items to be packed, and therefore at the very front of the lorry. "No matter, I must see the picture". We are not to be released from the pound until the picture is checked.

Dad and I are discussing how we should approach this, when from an office a few hundred feet away appear two official looking characters carrying some tape and a small box. "It is lunch-time now and we must seal your loading doors until we return in two hours time. Then we will expect you to unload the lorry and show us the picture". The doors are taped, an official seal is affixed to the tape and the officials are gone. There is not a lot that we can do in a Customs' pound so we head for the nearest café and order some lunch.

It is now just past six o'clock and having left the Port of Calais (vowing never to return), our next challenge is to find the delivery address. I take a right hand turn, ending up on the left of the road and bumper to bumper with a French lorry heading for the docks. "You stupid English" is heard beautifully pronounced as we again turn right, this time in to the courtyard of our destination.

I haven't been involved in the construction industry for too long, but can recognise a building site when I see one. Several piles of building materials surround us, scaffold poles, fencing, and a range of untidy sheds where it would seem the workers relax. The address scrawled on the delivery note is 'Flat 907'. To be honest I wouldn't have guessed that the partly completed building in front of us was either particularly safe, or nine storeys high, but I was wrong, because it was and our destination was on the top floor. I presume that the installation of the lifts is one of the last jobs to be done because there aren't any. Access is via a dangerous looking set of concrete stairs devoid of any handrails, and with a seventy-foot drop as we reach the top.

We are back home now, having missed two ferries and spending a cold night sleeping in the cab of the lorry, but to look on the bright side...

Episode 5

When I left Stanmore almost six years ago I promised my self that I would do everything that was available to me as life is so very precious. Many polio victims that I have met, and will meet in the future, have an inner force that drives us onwards. We are a determined group of people with a zest for life and all that it throws at us. We have beaten the virus (many of us take with us constant reminders of the battle), and through this battle have developed a force of mind and will power that drives us to achieve the almost unachievable.

I am constantly conscious of my physical appearance and aware of my limitations but this only forces me to try harder.

The decision to take the HGV driving course and subsequent test was, I suspect, an attempt to prove to myself that anything is possible. This was again the motive when I decided to take gliding lessons with a large well-established gliding club near Eastbourne. I would leave home at about seven o'clock in the morning, travel thirty miles to the club and then sit in the clubs' meeting room, sometimes all day, waiting for the weather to clear. But what a sensational feeling when eventually we were airborne. Standing ready at the top of a long hill, the glider is launched by a winch way below us to lift us high into the air, when with a tug of the release cable, we are free and alone. The sky is crystal blue, and the landscape is laid out neatly below us. We can see for miles. The only sound is the wind as we glide around seeking pockets of warm air to maintain or increase our height, or as we slowly wind our way back to earth to a graceful landing.

I loved it, I wanted more and more, but the costs, travel and unreliability of the weather gradually took their toll and I had to cease the sport.

I was married in the month of July in 1972 and before it ended in divorce twelve years later we had three wonderful sons. I instantly became a single parent and whilst trying to maintain full employment was mother and father to all three. They were hard times, difficult times, exhausting times, and great fun, and my feelings of satisfaction and achievement as I look at the three lovely young men today is immense.

There is an entire lifetime built around the period when I was a single parent father, and maybe in a future book I will express my thoughts and memories as I am today.

Taking to the air is too expensive and yet I want to be able to undertake a hobby that is both rewarding spiritually, but also physically, so my decision to purchase an ex-lifeboat recently converted to a sea-going fishing boat would seem to fit the bill completely. I can't swim, but with life jackets and buoys this needn't be a concern. The boat has a mud mooring in the middle of one of the fastest flowing rivers in the UK, and access is at specific heights of tide by a small powered dinghy housed on the quayside. The form of attack is to launch the dinghy in a heading approximately two hundred yards up or down river according to the direction of the tide. With full throttle on the outboard and the drift of the tide, we arrive about in line with our anchor point and reach out to grab the passing line attached to the stern of the boat. This manoeuvre forces the dinghy to swing round in line and tuck in behind the boat. For much of the time.

Miss the connection point and it is head for the opposite bank, walk up or down as required, dragging the dinghy, and then re-

launch. Sometimes this would require
several attempts.

Re-mooring the boat after a days fishing
expedition would require a similar
approach. With the need to approach the
mooring at speed, aim for the mooring buoy,
grab the line, preventing yourself being
pulled out of the boat and into the river
by the force of the sudden stop, and if all
fails, do it again.

This particular Sunday morning is blowing a
heavy gale with gusts of force nine
predicted at the harbour entrance. This has
the affect of producing a formidable wall
of churning sea usually up to six feet high
across the entrance as the storm tossed sea
in the channel meets the rushing tide
trying to escape the harbour. My newly
pregnant wife, and an old school friend and
her husband have suggested that perhaps we
could motor down the river and watch (from
a safe distance), this natural phenomenon.
We have arrived at our planned viewpoint
and the sight is truly spectacular. The
wind is blowing a good force eight and we
are finding it very difficult to stand on
deck. The sea in the channel some one
hundred yards away is in torment; it is a
mass of water in a filthy shade of grey
with long white rollers capping each angry
wave as they try to get through the harbour
entrance. I decide that I have seen enough
and start the engine, moving slowly forward
towards the entrance so that I could safely

turn back towards our mooring up river. Disaster has struck with the snapping of the throttle cable linkage from the controls to the engine housed down in the bilge of the boat. Without power the boat is being carried by the outgoing tide into the rapidly developing sea wall. I am screaming for my wife to lift of the engine cover while I try and steer the drifting boat away from the harbour entrance whilst praying that the engine does not stall. No good, the howling wind and increasing roughness of the sea is preventing my wife from lifting the cover, so dropping everything I raise the cover my self and by using the engines carburettor bring the engines to full power, and we move forward. My friend by this time has grasped how serious the situation is and has taken control of the wheel and by swinging around to full starboard, narrowly avoiding colliding with the stone harbour wall itself, we slowly gain ground and begin heading up river to safety.

We were the only people on the river that day, and within a few minutes there were none.

We did have many enjoyable times on the boat and in the time that we were proud owners we had not one accident or injury. We did have a couple of other misadventures though; the first was about five weeks after the cable incident.

Every year, Shoreham Airport hold their annual air display and today we have decided to watch the display from the comfort of our boat whilst moored just off the airport perimeter. Sandwiches are made and packed and with the same two friends as before we board the boat and head up river to find an ideal vantage spot. Within the hour we have anchored and am enjoying the display of aircraft and flying displays, many of which are passing right over our heads. It is a long day and yet before we realise it the displays are over and it is time for us to raise anchor and head back.

We lift the anchor, stowing it carefully away for next time, begin the engines, and at this stage I wonder why we are not moving. The tide has come in, we have drifted onto a sandbank, and the tide is now going out, rapidly. I suggest that we could, perhaps, rock the boat off the bank, but this is to no avail. We have water, but just not enough and the tide is continuing to go out. Wading to the bank is considered and dismissed after seeing the depth of mud we would have to wade through, so we need a plan B. I suddenly remember that our dinghy is attached at the stern and we could get back to the quay side in this. Ladies first of course, followed by friend and then the captain last, but as my friend left the boat, I could feel it move slightly towards the main channel. With a large rolling movement the boat without the major part of its load had found sufficient depth to refloat and was drifting down river towards our mooring. Restarting the engines and towing my passengers back to our mooring was not the ideal way to finish the day, but we were safe and dry.

I love sea fishing and the boat gave us many opportunities to go out into the Channel for a day, about three or four miles offshore, where we could catch some excellent fish.

This afternoon we had have had a very successful catch, with Bass, Plaice, Flounders, loads of Mackerel and a couple of Pollack and rounding into the harbour entrance I can see a dredger working to one side of the harbour channel. The boat is displaying an attractive array of different coloured flags and some of the men on deck begin waving to us. My friends and I wave back of course. There is the sound of a horn blasting, and continuing my way into the harbour I am now parallel with the dredger and about sixty feet away. Suddenly the men on deck are signalling to us to get out of the way and to move forward as fast as we can. I am completely at a loss as to why they are referring to us, but do as they say and move quickly forward. The steel cable was about four inches in diameter and came up out of the water like a cheese wire, vibrating to a halt showering water as it did so. The cable was approximately ten feet above our heads and no more than two feet from the stern of our boat.

Had we been slower or seven or so feet further back, the cable would have cut our boat in half like slicing through a ripe cheese. The dredger was working its way from side to side in the harbour entrance and using two guide cables attached to each side of the channel to pull it self broadside across whilst clearing the bed of silt.

Shortly afterwards I sold the boat and dinghy and swore never again.

I have always been a keen outdoor type of person and love to watch 'The Good Life' on television. The thought of being fully self-sufficient inspires me to enquire about renting a small parcel of woodland close to where I live. I am lucky and one of the local landowners is prepared to rent me two acres of land next door to a riding stables located off a quite lane about five mile from home.

One of the conditions set down by the owner is that I must completely enclose the plot with a reasonable quality fence as there are several people with gaming rights within the remainder of the woodland and a definite boundary must be maintained. I purchase rolls of wire mesh fencing and hundreds of fence posts and start about erecting the boundary. I am fully employed now by a local company so my time is limited, but every weekend is spent fence erecting until eventually the work is finished. I decide that we must have power and water on the site so this is arranged with the local statutory undertakings, and I purchase a second-hand beach-hut which will be the site hut.

Hours and hours are spent laying down tons of rubble to form a drive in to the site and I manage to install a line of lights to guide the way during the long winter nights.

Stock; we needed to stock our plot with some animals, but the choice was difficult until we heard that my excema could be eased by drinking goat's milk and other produce such as the curd and solid cheeses. Several of my wife's friends mentioned that they too would purchase the milk and cheese, so the hunt was on.

Scouring the local newspapers we read an advertisement for the sale of a young nanny goat not too far away and within the hour we are on our way. The address is down a long unmade track opening on to a range of near derelict buildings laughingly called a farm, where a range of very unhappy animals can be seen scratching around for food. The owner, a miserable looking man in a scruffy overcoat and wellingtons greets us and we are directed to a small paddock to one side of the main building. She is lovely; the sweetest looking goat that we have ever seen and we immediately fall in love with her. A deal is made and I make arrangements to collect her next weekend.

According to the farming magazines that we read, electric fencing is the latest method of keeping in stock and guided by the articles, I purchase and install a small paddock of electric fencing on a corner of our plot.

It is the weekend at last and after emptying our small Renault van we head off to collect our goat.
I suppose I should have suspected something was wrong at our first visit, but we were so taken by the nanny that all common sense had been forgotten. Apparently the nanny was only part of the package which also included a fierce looking Billy. His horns were knurled and twisted with one end missing (probably in a fight), and the smell was appalling. Still we had made a deal, and the nanny we wanted, so we bundle both goats into our tiny van and head home. Goats, like most animals, have one major reaction when frightened or distressed, and these were no exception. The Billy completely disgraces himself several times, but by the look on his face, doesn't give a damn. The nanny is a lot more refined but just as frightened.

It has taken us a horrendous hour and a half to reach the land and driving into our entrance I am pleased to see our neighbour, the stable manager, waiting by the gate.

He has looked at our goat enclosure and on seeing the Billy a shy grin begins to form on his face. "Do you intend keeping the Billy in there?" glancing towards the enclosure, "You do, well I'm not so sure that that is a good idea. Still it's your decision" Slightly put off by this remark, I lead the goats by their collars, open the enclosure gate and let them wander into their new home.

It has taken three minutes for the Billy to weigh up the electric fence, locate the weakest point, and with horns down clear the fence in one leap. The nanny on the other hand is pleased to see him go, and begins munching into a bag of fresh hay.

It is two hours later, and tired and filthy dirty, our neighbour and I have rounded up the Billy. We have tried to calm the many people that he attempted to mount, and are staking him to the ground with a length of rope that even King Kong would have found it difficult to escape from.

He lasted two days, the smell was unbearable, he continually charged anyone who attempted to go anywhere near him, and he had begun chewing his way through the rope. His departure in the back of a truck heading for slaughter was full of mixed emotions, most of them relief.

Our nanny is a dream, she has produced two lovely kids, (she was pregnant when we bought her), gallons of fresh milk and my excema has cleared.

Chickens are next and very soon we have two hundred free range chickens laying over one hundred and fifty large brown eggs every day. The problem is collecting the eggs every morning on the way to work. The chickens need a series of nesting boxes where they can lay their eggs for easy collection, so over the next few weekends I build a smart new chicken house with shelved nesting boxes and areas where the hens can roost at night if they wish. I also purchased a cockerel to keep the hens amused. Rasputin is evil. He sees every human as a potential enemy and guards his hens as fiercely as a Sheikh would guard his harem. It takes skilful planning and the patience of Job to outwit him, and every visit to collect the eggs becomes a battle of wits and sheer determination. I didn't always win and Rasputin would retreat with a conqueror stride on many an occasion. The eggs can wait until tomorrow.

Having built a very sound, spacious, warm, dry, and comfortable, series of nesting boxes, complete with feeders, etc., the design and construction of which I painstakingly followed from an 'expert' in poultry, I would often just set about waiting for the eggs to be produced!

This morning still employed full-time as a building surveyor I arrive at our site to feed and check on the live-stock, and of course, collect the eggs, before going on to work.

I think the main problem is that the chickens have not read the same books as I, and have decided to lay their eggs (almost 180 or so a day at the moment), anywhere but in the net boxes. It is surprising how difficult it is to find new laid brown eggs in an area of 2 acres of woodland, particularly so when it is pouring with rain.

This particular morning I think we are probably having one of our heaviest downpours, and it is still 'chucking' it down as I enter the 'so called' nest box. I have collected about 150 eggs and have decided to take advantage of the dry, very welcoming, hen house for a short spell.

I will never know, or understand, why I do what I do next. Without thinking, noticing that the roof of the hen house has begun to sag under the weight of the over night rainfall, (probably aggravated by a mountain of fallen leaves, etc.,), I reach up with my arm and gently lift the roof to throw off the water.

Water, as you may know, weighs 1 Tonne per cubic metre, and with the leaves and other debris, the gross weight that descended on me through the hole in the roof as my arm disappeared skywards, was potentially fatal. This did not include the eggs that I drop in the panic.

Needless to say there are no hens in the house at the time, they are probably under a series of trees and bushes, enjoying every minute. It takes a while for me to recover from the shock, and several weeks to repair the damage. I am also late for work.

The 'Good Life' continues with the introduction of six piglets bought from a friendly pig-farmer just up the road from us and these are installed in another corner of our plot with a sty made from old straw bales. Very warm and comfortable it is too. The plan is to fatten up the piglets as free range, and then have them slaughtered at the correct weight for pork. I have arranged a deal whereby the local slaughterhouse will prepare the meat into joints, and swap two of our pork pigs for two bacon pigs in lieu of any payment.

The difficulties come when it is time to load the pigs into the trailer ready for the journey. Pigs are very smart and highly intelligent and it didn't take them long to work out that the trailer ride was not for them. I have formed a tight passage from the sty to the trailer using straw bales and am carefully guiding the pigs towards the ramp. I didn't hear the signal, but as one, all six pigs cleared the bales and stood panting and staring at us some fifty yards away. It is time for plan B. This involves chasing each pig individually round and round the compound until one of us is exhausted. Hopefully it is the pig, whereby he is dragged unceremoniously into the trailer.

Shortly after this, our neighbour farmer who had helped us with the pigs gave up farming and move away to become a tree surgeon. I suspect that we may have had some influence on his decision. We also decide that pigs are not for us and concentrate on our chickens and goats.

The woodland that we rent comprises mainly Dutch Elm and many of these have become dangerously unstable, so with our young family running around, I decide to fell a few of the more dangerous ones. I purchase a second-hand petrol driven chain saw, read the manual, and begin felling the first. I cut a horizontal groove into the back of the tree about four feet of the ground in the opposite direction to where I want the tree to fall. Then gingerly begin to form a 'V' shaped cut on the front face of the tree just below the horizontal cut. I didn't hear the dreadful cracking sound, only that of my wife shouting at me to get out of the way. I manage to get ten feet or so from the tree, still carrying the chain saw. With an almighty thud the tree slides vertically along the 'V' cut and buries the sawn end into the ground only two feet from where it started, ending up perfectly upright, as if it had never moved. Now what, there is absolutely no way that I am going to get near the tree now, as it could fall in any direction, at any moment. Ropes are the answer, and my wife and I pass a rope around the back of the tree, and begin walking away from the tree in opposite directions.

The rope is drawn tight and with an equal pull the tree is felled to fall between us. The impact as it hits the ground, fills the air with masses of broken branches, leaves, debris and clouds of choking dust from decades of decay and uncultivated scrub. But it is down and safe.

I am getting quite good at this now, and the last one to do today is close to the road, so we have decided to ask some friends of ours to stand in the road to stop any traffic that may pass along as the tree falls, just in case.

The horizontal cut is made and I am completing the final 'V' cut away from the road. I warn my friends to stop the traffic and with my back to the road begin driving a wedge into the horizontal slot. The noise is deafening and it takes me only a split second to realise that something is wrong. The tree trunk where I have been cutting is hollow in the middle, and as the wedge is driven in the entire tree begins to collapse downwards. The wedge is forced out of the slot like an arrow, and with an ear-splitting crack the tree begins to fall towards the road. My friends frantically try to convince an irate car driver that it will be safer to stop where she is. Suddenly through the thick undergrowth and several smaller trees, the Elm crashes down on to the road, bouncing as it hits the tarmac. Smaller branches are thrown in every direction until it comes to a halt with a deadly hush. Everyone is stunned.

Episode 6

During the late 1980's I was working as a free-lance building surveyor which enabled me to base my working day around my children and allow me the opportunity to generate sufficient income for the annual holiday, running a car, etc.

On this particular morning I have been asked to carry out a building survey for a friend of a friend living in a large detached house to the north of our town. Entering the spacious lounge area it is easy to imagine that my client had a serious interest in flying as on almost every wall hung photographs of magnificent aircraft. May of these aircraft dated a few years ago, but some were more up to date and included the very latest in airliners.

Once I had completed the survey, and we returned to the lounge for a coffee, the conversation was directed towards the photographs. It transpired that my client had been a pilot for one of the large airlines and having recently retired was presently the Chief Flying Instructor at my local airfield. Naturally my imagination switched to overdrive and within a few minutes a deal had been struck. I was to begin a course of flying lessons on a single engined Cessna aircraft.

I could hardly wait, but eventually the pre-arranged day came around. The weather was good and we would start today.

I have been in a plane before, and had a trial flight in a helicopter at one of our local air-shows, but I am amazed at how cramped it is inside the Cessna. As a passenger I am sitting in the right hand seat, the ground checks have been made, the engine is powered up and we gather speed whilst running along the grass runway. Sixty knots and my instructor pulls back gently on the joystick and we are airborne. The ground is rapidly falling away as we climb up in to the clear blue sky. The noise is deafening, but the view sensational. Everything below us is as if made by skilled toy-maker. Each piece immaculately prepared and placed in exactly the right position. Trees, bushes, hedges, tiny animals and people, buildings of every shape and description laid out below in neat rows, each with a small garden, some with a brightly coloured car parked in the front driveway, the golden sun glinting off the roofs. Within minute we are at two thousand feet and flying parallel to the shoreline below. I can see the waves gently breaking on to the seashore and crowds of excited children splashing in the warm water. Some are building sandcastles.

We are now flying along a valley between two large clouds and we twist and turn in and out of the 'hills' on either side. We are climbing above them now and below us is a sea of soft billowing white down, through which I can glimpse the occasional speck of blue or green from the land below. I am lost in a world of dreams, floating on air, with the vivid blue summer sky high above us. Banking to one side, it is time to return and we head towards the airfield. The plane has dual controls and asked to take control I can feel the force of the plane as it falls slowly downward. I am too 'heavy' on the stick and the plane is tossed about like a ship in a high sea. "Be gentle with her" I am advised, and soon grasp that I need very little movement on the stick to produce changes of direction or rate of climb. I am told to use my feet on the rudder controls and can feel the 'crab like' movement that an incorrect rudder position can create. "Don't forget to increase the power slightly, or dip the nose when banking or we will lose height. Increase the power when climbing to avoid a stall" There is a lot to remember and it will take a while to get use to the controls, but the experience of it all is wonderful. My instructor completes the landing and we roll gently to a halt. I will be back next week for lesson two.

Every person intending to take the controls of an aircraft must first apply to the Aviation Authority for a medical certificate confirming that you are fit and able to operate a plane safely. The concern, I believe, is that you must not be a hazard to either other aircraft, or people on the ground. I am not sure that the safety of the pilot is under consideration. My present medical condition does not lend itself to achieving an A1 grade, but I am distinctly anxious when I arrive at the surgery of the approved Medical Officer. A brief history of my past illnesses, some discussion about the spinal fusion, and an intake of breath when discovering that I have only one good lung doesn't ease the anxiety. However, concluding a considerable number of tests, I am declared fit enough to fly a single or double-engined aircraft, but for pleasure purposes only. A commercial licence is out of the question.

Armed with my new certificate I arrive at the airfield a week later and lesson two begins. Take off is a reasonably straightforward manoeuvre once I get to grips with the rudder controls which whilst on the ground operates the small pilot wheel at the front of the plane. The first few take offs resemble my golf game where I tend to explore the entire fairway and surrounding land rather than head in a single straight line to the pin. A four hundred-yard hole and I probably walk at least eight hundred before the green is reached. Drunk and disorderly is probably a good way of summing up my initial attempts to reach the sky.

Once breaking contact with Mother Earth, my instant reaction is to pull hard on the joy-stick placing us in an almost vertical position and forcing shouts of "What the hell are you doing" from my dear old white haired instructor. Once I master this and climb steadily to eight hundred feet, I raise the flaps a couple of notches and continue climbing until we reach eleven hundred feet, which is the approach height for this airfield. A tight bank to the North, continue up for a further nine hundred feet or so, and then begin to level off. Easy. I always wonder why my instructor looks behind when we have just left the ground. It's too late to pickup something that I may have dropped!

Level flight is remarkably easy. Keeping a close eye on the controls whilst listening to the control tower and looking around for near traffic becomes automatic, and at times I can actually take in the view. "Okay, lets try a landing" from my instructor and my palms begin to sweat and beads of perspiration appear on my forehead, and strangely the guy in the next seat. I reduce my height to eleven hundred feet, and line up the plane for an approach. Check with air traffic control that I have permission to land, look for any near traffic, and reduce height to eight hundred feet whilst maintaining a straight flight with the rudder. This is becoming frighteningly complicated and I am finding it difficult to know what to do next. At 100 Knots the ground is coming up rather quicker than I had hoped. "If you don't want to kill us both, I would suggest that you cut the engines, lower the flaps, and level off until the speed is down to sixty knots, but don't stall it". Confidence, that's just what I wanted. Oh well, in for a dollar, in for a pound, I cut the engines, level off the plane and stare at the speedometer. "Peter", I don't like the sound of this, "You have missed the runway by about half a mile, if you land now, we shall be in the river. Go round and try again". On the television this sounds fairly simple and the pilot react without any obvious signs of concern. With me it is different and to be honest, if I could get out and walk from here, I probably would. "Increase the power, raise the flaps, gain height and go around for a second attempt."

The second time round and for some reason I am in control, and following handbook style manoeuvres I land the aircraft and taxi to the parking area. "Well done, that was really good. See you next week ". I'm not sure.

I have had over thirty-five hours of training including endless 'touch and go's'. This is where the aircraft is landed on the runway, but does not stop, and instead immediately takes off for a further flight. The object is to just touch the runway, avoid leaving too much of the undercarriage behind and repeat this several times to practice the landing and take off techniques.

Today I feel good, confident and am looking forward to my flight. Ground checks are completed, control tower notified and I taxi to the runway awaiting clearance to take off. My instructor is wearing a broad grin. "Well, Peter, I think it is time for your first solo flight. I will meet you in the club bar and you can buy me a drink. Good luck, you'll be fine" With a pat on my shoulder he steps out of the plane and walks back to the hangers.

The control tower are asking me to either take off or vacate the runway so I take a deep breath, whisper a short prayer to whoever is listening, and accelerate down the runway. Sixty knots, lower the flaps, increase power, raise the nose and I'm airborne. Watch my rate of ascent, keep straight, control the rudder, keep an eye on my speed, and begin to level off at eleven hundred feet. Come round to the

North, climb to two thousand feet and level off completely. Trim back the power, and relax. Exploring the view I can see my car parked next to the hanger, club members are having a quiet drink under colourful umbrellas on the patio, and the ground seems a long way away.

Time to notify control of my intention to request approach, and I receive the go ahead. Bring the aircraft around, watch my speed and elevation, notify control, line up the runway and begin my approach. Height is fine, speed is fine. I keep forgetting the rudders so am coming in like a demented crab. If I land in this position I will roll the plane. Straighten the rudder, cut power, raise the nose, lower flaps, and continue on line. The ground is coming up. I can see the line marking the centre of the runway. It looks good. Speed good, rudder good, ascent good. Twenty feet to touchdown. At the last moment I flare the plane, and feel the judder as the wheels make contact with Mother Earth. The drink tastes really good. I have flown solo and live to tell the tale.

Episode 7

There are some parts of life that I have chosen to forget. Maybe one day I shall put the proverbial pen to paper and document some more episodes, but in the meantime my life has changed. I am a lecturer in a local College of Further Education, lecturing in the very subjects that carried me through many financially difficult years whilst single handed bringing up my three sons. I enjoy the many experiences very much and have a wealth of anecdotes to be shared with you at a later date. I developed a wide range of friends and colleagues. These are not only within the College, but many of the students who pass through our lectures return to show us how they have progressed, some raising a family of their own.

Life, however, is unpredictable, and like so many polio survivors of the 50's and 40's, the very cause of our determination and endurance is returning to haunt us all. During the last five years or so I have noticed deterioration in many of my physical abilities. Excessive tiredness and exhaustion, a weakening of various muscles, difficulties in swallowing and breathing, particularly when tired, and a general feeling of despondency. Anger, frustration, depression, these are the feelings that most of us are sensing at the moment. The enemy has returned and in force. The 'normal' living of life over the last forty or so, years has taken its toll and the already damaged nerve endings are beginning to weaken.

'Post Polio Syndrome', or 'The Late Effects of Polio' is trying to complete what the initial Polio virus failed to accomplish those many years ago. We weren't defeated then, and we won't be defeated now. Life will go on, and I will continue to experience many wonderful events throughout the next fifty years. Some will be joyful, some sorrowful, but all of them not to be missed.

Good luck with every one of your endeavours, and may your God be with you.

Peter

About the Author

Peter Thwaites is a Polio survivor from the early 1950's and has a wealth of experiences to relate from his birth and the onset of Polio to the present day as a college lecturer. Peter is a qualified Building Surveyor and has a Masters Degree in Land Information Management and Mapping. He has been published in several professional magazines on subjects as Geographical Information Systems, and Facilities Management.. He lectures on professional aspects of the construction industry, in particular: Building Law, CAD, Building and Topographical Surveying, and Planning, He is a single parent father and has three sons.

www.ingramcontent.com/pod-product-compliance
Lightning Source LLC
Chambersburg PA
CBHW030355290526
45785CB00004B/1754